Modeling Cancer

John A. Allocca, D.Sc., Ph.D.

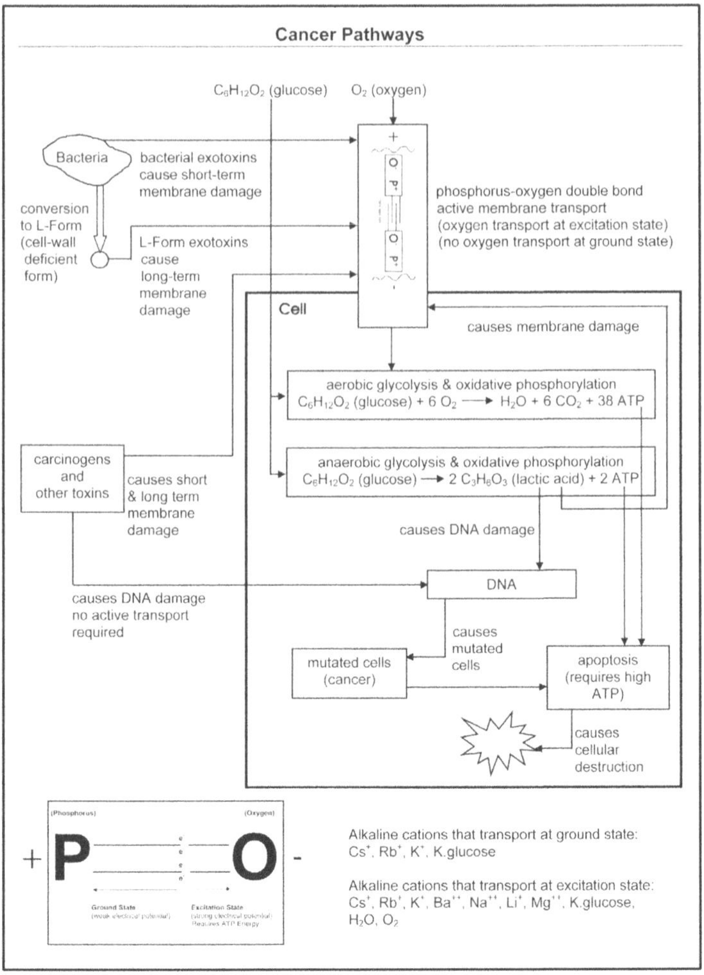

Modeling Cancer

John A. Allocca, D.Sc., Ph.D.

Published by
Allocca Biotechnology, LLC
19 Lorraine Court
Northport, New York 11768
Phone (631) 757-3919
john@allocca.com
www.allocca.com

ISBN 978-0976921356

Library of Congress Control Number: 2010911925

Table of Contents

Chapter 1 - What Can Cause Cancer?

The cell membrane becomes damaged from bacterial exotoxins, other toxins, and carcinogenic substances.

When the cell membrane is damaged, it switches from excitation state mode to ground state mode.

When the cell membrane is in the ground state mode, it cannot transport oxygen.

When there is not enough oxygen in the cell, energy is produced by anaerobic glycolysis whereby only 2 ATP molecules and lactic acid are produced per cycle vs 38 ATP molecules and water per cycle with aerobic glycolysis.

Consequently, lactic acid builds up inside of the cell further damaging the cell membrane and damaging the DNA.

There is not enough ATP energy with anaerobic glycolysis to activate apoptosis. Apoptosis is a cell's self-destruct mechanism.

The reproduction of damaged cells and DNA is the reason the body ages, organs degrade, and cancer begins.

Accumulated toxins damage cell membranes and DNA when detoxification systems do not adequately function.

Detoxification systems and apoptosis may not function if adequate oxygen and other chemical substances are not transported through the cell membranes into the cells.

A weak or overwhelmed immune system may not remove the cancer cells from the body.

Chapter 2 - Toxins, Detoxification, and Disease

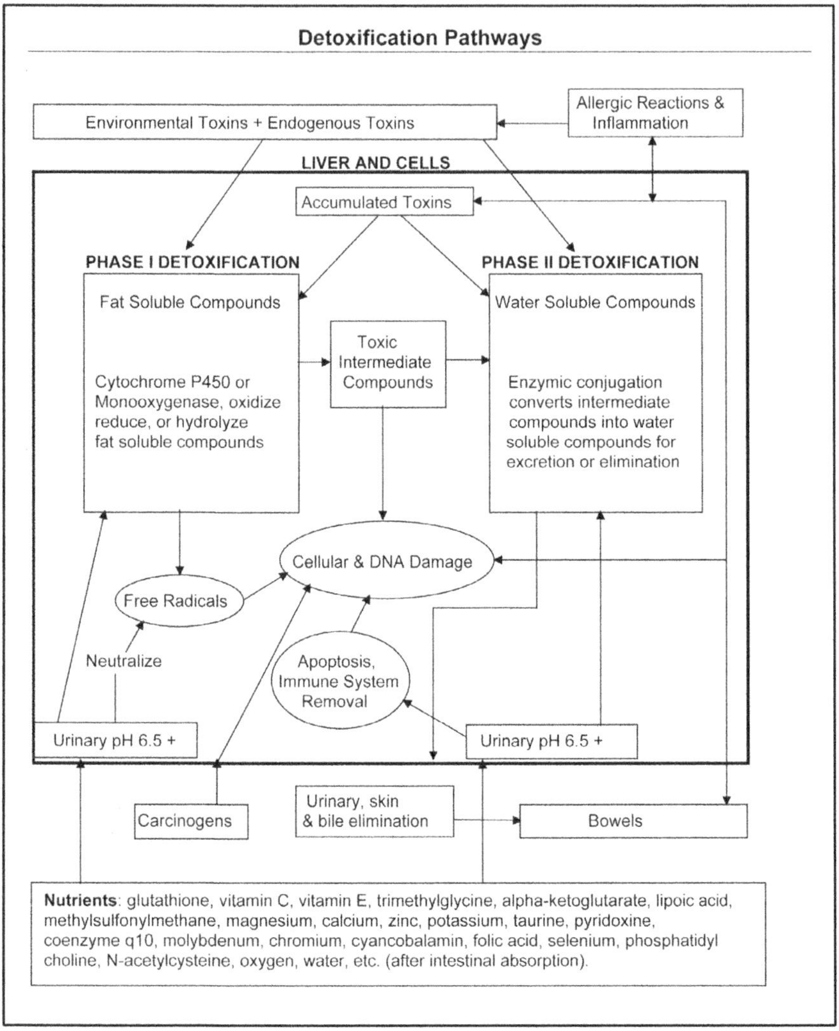
Detoxification Pathways
Environmental Toxins + Endogenous Toxins
Allergic Reactions & Inflammation
LIVER AND CELLS
Accumulated Toxins
PHASE I DETOXIFICATION
Fat Soluble Compounds
Cytochrome P450 or Monooxygenase, oxidize reduce, or hydrolyze fat soluble compounds
Toxic Intermediate Compounds
PHASE II DETOXIFICATION
Water Soluble Compounds
Enzymic conjugation converts intermediate compounds into water soluble compounds for excretion or elimination
Cellular & DNA Damage
Free Radicals
Neutralize
Apoptosis, Immune System Removal
Urinary pH 6.5 +
Urinary pH 6.5 +
Carcinogens
Urinary, skin & bile elimination
Bowels
Nutrients: glutathione, vitamin C, vitamin E, trimethylglycine, alpha-ketoglutarate, lipoic acid, methylsulfonylmethane, magnesium, calcium, zinc, potassium, taurine, pyridoxine, coenzyme q10, molybdenum, chromium, cyancobalamin, folic acid, selenium, phosphatidyl choline, N-acetylcysteine, oxygen, water, etc. (after intestinal absorption).

Damage to the cells from toxins is the major cause of many health problems. Toxicity from foreign chemicals (exotoxins) can cause damage to almost all cells of the body. Symptoms include: fatigue, headaches, neurological disorders, chemical sensitivities, immune dysfunction, and liver disorders. Food is often a major source of toxins. There are thousands of chemicals used by the food industry during processing and packaging. Many farmers use pesticides, which are passed along to us. In addition to these external sources of toxins, the body also produces toxins internally called, endotoxins resulting from digestion, immune system functions, stress, etc. Endotoxins may also be produced as the result of allergies and sensitivities.

Increased intestinal permeability (leaky gut syndrome) can allow exotoxins to be absorbed into the blood stream along with antigens and microorganisms. Candida albicans overgrowth can cause an imbalance in the intestinal microflora (dysbiosis) and offset the immune response of the intestinal tract. Candida albicans can change to the mycel form and penetrate the intestinal wall, leaving behind microscope holes in the intestinal wall. Candida albicans also produce toxins called aldehydes. Supplementation with probiotics such as lactobacillus acidophilus and lactobacillus bifidus is important to keep candida albicans under control and maintain a balanced intestinal flora.

Congestive bowel toxicity can greatly increase the amount of toxins produced in the gastrointestinal track.

How does the body deal with toxins? Fat-soluble toxins are easily absorbed but poorly excreted. Often, they accumulate in the body and cause damage to tissues and organs. Fat-soluble chemicals are converted to water-soluble chemicals, primarily in the liver, and in some cells, in a two-step process so that the water soluble toxins can be excreted by the urine, liver, and skin. The skin is a vitally important organ that eliminates toxins through perspiration.

During the first phase of detoxification, fat-soluble chemicals are converted into intermediate chemicals. As a result of this process, free radicals are also produced. The free radicals and the intermediate chemicals can cause damage to the cells. Adequate antioxidants must be present to detoxify these intermediate compounds produced during the first phase of detoxification. The first phase may also detoxify some chemicals directly without requiring a second phase conversion.

During the second phase, the intermediate chemicals are converted into water-soluble, chemicals, which are less toxic and easily excreted in the urine, bile, and skin.

It is now obvious why it is so important to avoid toxic chemicals from the environment. Drink uncontaminated water. Tap water should be filtered to remove lead, chlorine, heavy metals, and bacteria. It is also important to have an adequate supply of anti-oxidants to prevention cellular damage.

The ability of the liver to detoxify is determined by the availability of the appropriate nutrients and enzymes. An adequate supply of antioxidants is vitally important after the first phase of converting fat-soluble toxins, which produce free radicals. Reduced glutathione, superoxide dismutase, and catalase are the primary antioxidants used in the body to neutralize free radicals. Other antioxidants include: beta-carotene, vitamin E, vitamin C, selenium, n-acetylcysteine, alpha lipoic acid, and proanthocyanidins (grape seed extract). Vitamin and mineral cofactors required for cytochrome P-450 reactions include: riboflavin, niacin, magnesium, iron, and other trace minerals. Phytochemicals such as indoles from cruciferous vegetables and quercetin also help during the first phase of detoxification.

Other second phase conjugating agents include: amino acids such as glycine, cysteine, glutamine, methionine, taurine, glutamic acid, and asparatic acid.

Vitamin, mineral, and protein deficiencies will decrease the activity of the detoxification pathways. Fats and omega 6 polyunsaturated oils can promote the uptake of many chemical carcinogens. Olive oil (monounsaturated) and omega 3 polyunsaturated oils (EPA, DHA) have a neutral effect in promoting the uptake of carcinogens.

Cruciferous vegetables such as broccoli, cauliflower, brussel sprouts, watercress, and cabbage enhance the first phase of detoxification.

Garlic and onions contain flavonoid compounds, such as quercetin, which diminish the mutation of many carcinogens.

Turmeric contains curcumin, which acts as an antioxidant and helps protect cells and DNA from free radical damage. Turmeric also acts as an anti-inflammatory agent.

As previously discussed, the detoxification process requires various nutrients to function. Without such nutrients in the cells, intermediate compounds can cause cellular and DNA damage. If the apoptosis system (cells self destruct if they are damaged) does not get the proper nutrients, the damaged cells can reproduce. If the immune system does not get the proper nutrients, the damaged cells can reproduce out of control causing cancer.

Getting the nutrients into the blood is only the first step. The nutrients must enter the cells in order to be available for use by the cells. In order for the nutrients to get into the cells, they must be transported though the cell membrane. When there is a lack of nutrients, particularly oxygen inside the cell, there is a build-up of lactic acid inside the cell. Excessive lactic acid damages the cell membrane transport mechanism and DNA. Lactic acid causes the cell to become acidic (lower pH). There is a weak correlation between intracellular pH and urine pH/saliva pH. A urine and/or saliva pH must be 6.5 or greater is an estimate of how the membrane transport mechanism may be functioning.

The Process of Aging and Disease

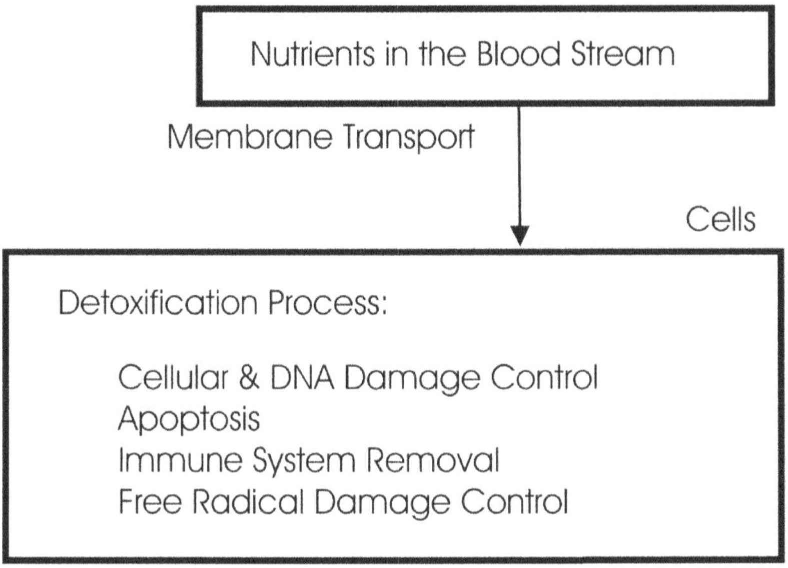

Nutrition and Membrane Transport Mechanisms

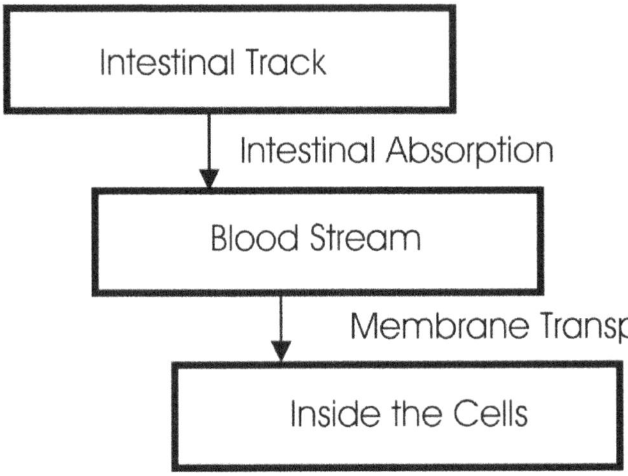

Chapter 3 - The Effects of Toxicity

Toxins occur in the surrounding environment and are produced internally. The body is designed to detoxify them, provided the body has an appropriate supply of chemicals (nutrients). The detoxification process converts fat-soluble toxins to water-soluble toxins, which are excreted. If they are not converted and excreted, toxins accumulate in the body, which eventually cause cellular DNA damage, aging, and disease.

Non-toxic food can also affect body chemistry and produce toxins. High in glycemic-index foods, such as sugar and starch will stimulate the body to produce too much insulin and cholesterol, which leads to inflammation, constricted blood vessels, pain, acidosis, and disease.

Acidosis is a condition whereby there is too much lactic acid in the cells, which eventually causes cellular and DNA damage. If the cells' DNA is damaged and the programmed cellular self-destruction mechanism, known as apoptosis, is not functioning properly, and the immune system does not remove the cell, it will reproduce. The continued reproduction of these DNA damaged cells becomes a cancerous tumor.

Chapter 4 - Sources of Toxins

Chemicals in Food

A great number of health problems can be attributed to a higher exposure to toxins than the body can detoxify. Toxicity from foreign chemicals (exotoxins) can cause damage to almost all organs of the body. Symptoms include fatigue, headaches, neurological disorders, chemical sensitivities, immune dysfunction, and liver disorders. Food is often the main source of toxins. The food industry uses approximately 3,000 chemicals during processing and approximately 12,000 chemicals in food packaging materials. Pesticides are found in 90% of foods.

Endotoxins

In addition to external sources of toxins, the body also produces endotoxins, which result from digestion, immune system functions, emotional stress, food allergies, sensitivities, etc.

Candida Albicans Overgrowth

Intestinal overgrowth of Candida albicans (yeast) is becoming a common problem. Diet is a critical component in the process of controlling Candida albicans overgrowth. Continuing research on Candida albicans overgrowth indicates that our lifestyles with diets high in sugars, widespread use of antibiotics (much of which is passed on to humans from the meat of farm animals that have been fed antibiotics), environmental pollution, stress, steroid drugs, and birth control pills along with the lack of acidophilus and bifidobacteria supplementation carries a lot of the blame for this persistent and growing health concern.

Candida albicans is a yeast-like fungus that is present in the stools, genitourinary tract, throat, and skin of normal people. An overgrowth of Candida albicans can occur in those whose normal defense mechanisms may have been weakened by underlying disease, antibiotic therapy or immunosuppressive agents or any other factors, which may weaken the immune system or intestinal flora.

Candida albicans normally resides in the intestinal tract along with E. coli, lactobacillus acidophilus, lactobacillus bifidus, enterococci, coliforms, etc., aiding in the digestion of food and the production of vitamins without causing harm, provided the bacteria and fungi are present in proper balance. The use of antibiotics and other bacteriostatic agents can destroy the bacterial flora of the intestinal tract without harming the yeast (Candida albicans). Without the presence of bacterial flora, Candida albicans can grow without control.

Once, overgrowth of Candida albicans has occurred in the intestinal tract, it forms myceles, which are spike-like structures that allow it to penetrate the intestinal walls and enter the bloodstream. The intestinal walls become damaged from the myceles leaving holes in the walls. After entering the blood, Candida albicans causes an inflammatory immune system response. Additionally, whole proteins and other large molecules can pass through the holes in the damaged intestinal walls, referred to as Increased Intestinal Permeability or Leaky Gut Syndrome, causing further allergic reactions to occur. It may take many years to repair the damage to the intestinal walls.

In the bloodstream, Candida albicans can mutate to a cell wall deficient form and "hide" from a weak immune system. In the cell wall deficient form there are no cell wall antigens to provoke an immune reaction with fever. It is possible to have systemic candidiasis for a lifetime if not properly treated. From the blood, Candida albicans will eventually invade the tissues and organs of the body, creating disease and malfunctions of various bodily systems.

In addition to Candidiasis, damage to the intestinal walls can occur from: using non-steroidal anti-inflammatory drugs (NSAID'S such as aspirin, ibuprofen, etc.), HIV infection, Lyme disease, intestinal infection, intestinal dysboisis, maldigestion, malabsorption, alcoholism, aging, deficient

IgA, giardiasis, ingestion of allergic foods, ingestion of offending chemicals, trauma, and endotoxima.

Allergic reactions may produce symptoms such as: fatigue, depression, chronic dermatological infections or rashes, acne, abdominal bloating, intestinal gas, indigestion, constipation or diarrhea, chemical sensitivities, food allergies, hypoglycemia, premenstrual tension, endometriosis, prostatitis, vaginitis, inability to concentrate, frequent mood shifts, rheumatoid arthritis, and loss of memory.

When a particular food causes an allergic reaction, a certain amount of pain is produced. The brain detects this pain and produces endorphins, which are similar to narcotics, to eliminate the pain. If the food is consumed regularly, the body will crave that food because it leads to the production endorphins. Similarly, Candidiasis will cause cravings for breads, wheat, sugars, starches, and yeast containing foods. These foods cause the Candida albicans to grow and stimulate allergic reactions. If sleepiness occurs after a meal, it is usually from an allergic reaction to the food or because the food was improperly combined. A great deal of discipline is required to avoid these foods.

Clinical Symptoms include: abdominal bloating, intestinal gas, Indigestion, constipation or diarrhea, chemical sensitivities, food allergies, hypoglycemia, premenstrual tension, endometriosis, prostatitis, vaginitis, chronic dermatological infections or rashes, acne, inability to concentrate, frequent mood shifts, loss of memory fatigue/

lethargy, depression, desire for refined carbohydrates or yeast containing foods. The most pronounced symptom of Candidiasis is chronic fatigue, especially after eating food or snacks that contain large amounts of sugar or simple carbohydrates. Often people get "sleepy" after such a meal or snack. Candida thrives on simple carbohydrates, especially sugar.

Clostridium and Other Bacterial Overgrowth

Recent research is indicating a complication of intestinal Candida albicans overgrowth, as a result of antibiotic therapy, with an associated intestinal overgrowth of the bacteria Clostridium difficile. There are also many bacteria that enter the stomach from the food supply. If an individual is experiencing stress, that individual may not produce enough hydrochloric acid to destroy microorganisms that enter the stomach from the food supply. Helicobacter pylori is a typical bacteria that invades the stomach and may eventually cause an ulceration in the stomach or intestinal lining and/or cancer.

In a recent small research investigation, the examination of blood revealed a significant reduction of Candida albicans, after the proper course of action, without a significant reduction of symptoms. In these cases, small amounts of unidentified bacillus bacteria were also seen in the blood. A comprehensive digestive stool analysis was performed, which revealed high fecal S-IgA, high leukocytes, and high red blood cells. Such results indicate a bacterial overgrowth. Clostridium difficile overgrowth is a common result of antibiotic therapy. Clostridium difficile produces two major toxins, named toxin A and toxin B. Toxin A mediates alteration in fluid secretion, enhances inflammation, and induces postcapillary venules to leak albumin. Toxin B inhibits ADP ribosylation of Rho proteins. Both toxins cause disruption and condensation of F actin, which results in electrophysiological alterations of colonic tissue. Some antibiotics trigger toxin production. Various components of bowel flora may suppress toxin production such as, Clostridium sordelli, which neutralize cytoxin B. When antibiotics destroy the more sensitive components of bowel flora, more resistant organisms may produce enzymes such a b-lactmases that can inactivate antibiotics and facilitate the growth of Clostridium difficile.

The symptoms of Clostridium difficile overgrowth are similar to that of Candida albicans overgrowth, and may include ulcerative colitis, anemia, and malabsorption. Ulcerative colitis can lead to weight loss. Malabsorption can lead to excessive eating and weight gain. In the cases with Clostridium difficile overgrowth, which was discovered after the course of action for Candida albicans overgrowth, success was finally achieved after a course of action for Clostridium difficile overgrowth.

A Candida IgG or IgE blood test and/or a comprehensive digestive stool analysis can indicate an overgrowth of candida albicans and other pathogens. A urinary indican test can indicate the level of intestinal dysbiosis.

Increased Intestinal Permeability

Increased intestinal permeability (leaky gut) is a major cause of food intolerance, sensitivity, and allergy. The small intestine is an organ that absorbs nutrients and acts as a barrier to toxic compounds and large molecules. Increased intestinal permeability is referred to as "leaky gut syndrome," which allows toxic compounds and large molecules to enter the lymphatic and blood system.

All material that passes through the intestinal mucosa is scrutinized by the immune system. It is here that the immune system may have it highest exposure to antigens. Increased intestinal permeability can allow large amounts of antigens to enter the systemic circulation were they may react with antibodies. If the antigens are similar to the body's own tissues, the resulting process may manifest itself as an autoimmune disease.

The lactulose and manitol urine test is used to measure the degree that the two simple sugars are absorbed into the body.

Increased intestinal permeability can be caused by: candida albicans overgrowth, non-steroidal anti-inflammatory drugs (NSAID's), HIV infection, intestinal infection, intestinal dysboisis, maldigestion, malabsorption, alcoholism, aging, deficient IgA, giardiasis, candidiasis, ingestion of allergic foods, ingestion of offending chemicals, and trauma and endotoxima.

Congestive Bowel Toxicity

Often the bowel is ignored as being associated with health disorders. Constipation is such a widespread problem that laxatives are one of the highest selling classes of drugs in this country. Imagine food sitting on a table decaying for weeks, months and even years. What will happen if this food is eaten? This is analogous to food that remains in the large intestines for the same length of time. Many of the decayed materials and toxins get into the blood stream and have an adverse effect on health.

Bacterial action plays a major role in nutrition and digestion. Friendly bacteria synthesize valuable nutrients by digesting portions of the fecal mass. Vitamin K, portions of the B-complex, and other vitamins are produced. Any remaining proteins are broken down by the bacterial and fungal flora. Other bacterial by products include: indole, skatole, hydrogen sulfide, fatty acids, methane gas, and carbon dioxide. The normal bacterial flora can easily be destroyed by antibiotics. Destruction of the bacterial flora in the intestinal tract can lead to the overgrowth of Candida albicans and Clostridium difficile in the intestines. The results are malabsorption of vitamins and consequently fatigue.

The time it takes for feces to be produced depends upon the amount of roughage and water content in the food. Bulkier feces travel faster because the bowel muscles can work on the material to move it. Soft, fiberless, feces become very difficult for the colon to move. The longer it takes to move, the more water is absorbed, making the feces compacted, hard and difficult to eliminate. Laxatives increase the amount of liquid retained in the feces and act as a lubricant. Laxatives may be combined with irritating substances. One can easily become dependent on laxatives that may destroy normal bowel function. Diarrhea (liquid feces) may be produced by excessive use of laxatives, nervous stress, infection, or the presence of toxic substances.

There are many diseases of the colon including: adhesion (caused by inflammations and irritations to the bowel wall), ballooning (caused by backed up feces), colitis and spastic bowel (irritable/overworked bowel which is highly associated with stress), diverticulosis (colon hernia caused by a diet lacking bulk or fiber), mucosal dysfunction (when the mucous lining becomes stagnant), stricture (narrowing of a passageway usually after colitis), ulceration (due to irritation, abrasions, infections and toxic concentrations). The American Cancer Society stresses the importance of high fiber diets to reduce the risk of colon cancer. Raw vegetables and fruits are best and fresh vegetable juice is excellent. White bread is very congestive and clogging.

An individual may move their bowels regularly, but may have material covering the lining of the colon (like a partially clogged water pipe).

Tyramine

Tyramine is a vaso-active amino acid that displaces norepinephrine from the nerve endings and epinephrine from the adrenal glands. Monoamine oxidase is in the gastrointestinal tract and inactivates tyramine. There is an adverse reaction when there is either too much tyramine or too little monoamine oxidase. The tyramine content in foods vary greatly due to different processing, aging, fermentation, ripening and/or contamination. Many foods that contain small amounts of tyramine develop large amounts of tyramine if the food products were left to spoil, age (not fresh), or fermented. The emphasis is placed on FRESH FOODS. Fruits that are permissible should be very fresh. Avoid leftovers kept in the refrigerator especially meats, dry packages mixes and can products (prepared foods), yeast extracts, and protein extracts. Remember, foods increase in their tyramine content as they age or ferment. For example, bananas are permissible if they are fresh, not if they are overripe.

Tyramine can also be produced by bacteria in the gastrointestinal track. Helicobactor pylori can produce large amounts of tyramine in the gut. Various bacteria in the gut can cause an increase in the production of tyramine.

Mild tyramine reactions can occur with approximately 6 mg of tyramine. Severe reactions can occur with 10-25 mg tyramine of tyramine.

Approximate tyramine contents of food:

Cheddar cheese = 1.5 mg/g (42.5 mg/ounce)
Blue Stilton = 0.2 mg/g (5.6 mg/ounce)
Gouda = 0.02 mg/g (0.56 mg/ounce)
Beer = 0.02 mg/g (0.56 mg/ounce)
Wine = 0.025 mg/g (0.71 mg/ounce)
Yeast Extracts = 2 mg/g (56.6 mg/ounce)

Tyramine Pathways

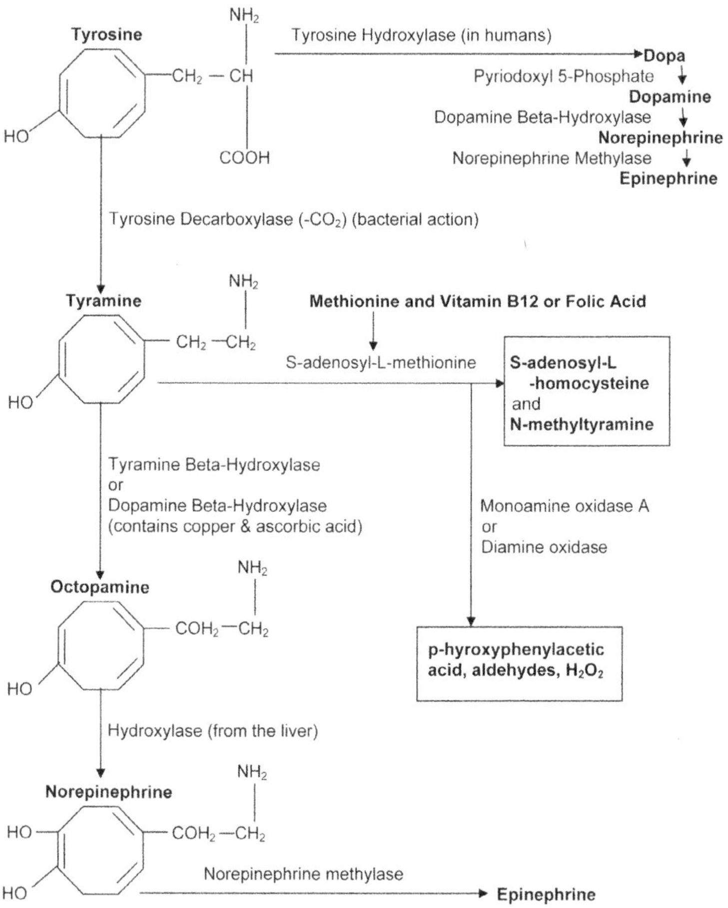

Tyramine is a potent vasoconstrictor and displaces neurotransmitters.
Octopamine is a potent vasoconstrictor in humans and neurotransmitter in insects.

Allergic Reactions

The antigen-antibody system is like a lock and key. An appropriately coded key must be made to fit in and turn the lock cylinder. Upon entry of a foreign antigen, the lymphoid tissue macrophages phagocytize the antigen and then present it to adjacent lymphocytes. Those lymphocytes specific for that antigen enlarge and become lymphoblasts and some differentiate to form plasmablasts, which are procursors to plasma cells.

The mature plasma cell then produces gamma globulin antibodies, which are secreted into the lymph and carried into the circulating blood. Some of the lymphoblasts form moderate numbers of new B lymphocytes similar to the original clone. They remain dormant in the lymphoid tissue and are called memory cells. Exposed to the same antigen they will elicit a much more rapid response.

Antibodies are gamma globulins called immunoglobulins and composed of light and heavy polypeptide chains. Antibodies can inactivate an invader in several ways:

Agglutination, in which multiple antigenic agents are bound together in a clump;

Precipitation, in which the complex of soluble antigen and antibody becomes insoluble and precipitates;

Neutralization, in which the antibodies cover the toxic sites of the antigenic agent; and

Lysis, in which very potent antibodies directly attack membranes of cellular agents and cause them to rupture.

Allergic tendency is a phenomenon that is passed on genetically and characterized by large quantities of antibodies called reagins or sensitizing antibodies. When the allergen enters the body, an allergen-reagin reaction takes place and subsequent allergic reaction. During the allergic reaction, mast cells and basophils burst releasing histamine and other inflammatory chemicals.

Hay fever is the allergen-reagin reaction that occurs in the nose. Histamine is released in response and causes local vasodilation and capillary permeability.

Asthma is the allergen-reagin reaction that occurs in the bronchioles of the lungs, which causes spasm of the bronchiolar smooth muscles.

IgA reactions occur on body surfaces and the gut.

IgD reactions are minor.

IgE (type I) reactions are immediate allergic reactions such as itching, hayfever and food allergies. There is an immediate release of histamine from the basophils.

IgM, IgG (type II, III, IV) reactions activate primary antibodies to tag or neutralize invaders. Type II reactions consist of food immune reactions. Type III reactions are more subtle than type II. Type IV reactions are often referred to as a delayed hypersensitivity reaction which may take 3 to 4 days to appear and 3 to 4 days to disappear. In some cases the reaction can last as long as 14 days. Only one molecule is required to start an immune reaction.

Allergic reactions may produce symptoms such as: fatigue, depression, chronic dermatological infections or rashes, acne, abdominal bloating, intestinal gas, indigestion, constipation or diarrhea, chemical sensitivities, food allergies, hypoglycemia, premenstrual tension, endometriosis, prostatitis, vaginitis, inability to concentrate, frequent mood shifts, rheumatoid arthritis, and loss of memory.

When a particular food stimulates an allergic reaction (inflammatory response), a certain amount of pain is produced. The brain detects this pain and produces endorphins, which are similar to narcotics, to eliminate the pain. If the food is consumed regularly, the body will crave that food because it leads to the production endorphins. Candida albicans overgrowth will cause cravings for breads, wheat, sugars, starches, and yeast containing foods. These foods cause the Candida albicans to grow and stimulate allergic reactions.

If sleepiness occurs after a meal, it is usually from an allergic reaction to the food or because the food was improperly combined. A great deal of discipline is required to avoid these foods.

Liver Toxicity

Detoxification takes place within the liver and within the cells. Most of the detoxification takes place within the liver. If the amount of nutrients that enter the liver and cells is less than the amount required to detoxify the toxin load, toxins will begin to accumulate leading to aging, organ degradation, and disease.

If the liver does not detoxify toxins, they will accumulate in the liver. Excess toxins in the liver may enter the blood stream and be transported throughout the body.

The liver is the major organ responsible for detoxifying toxins produced in the body and environmental toxins. To do this, it must have an adequate supply of nutrients. The liver excretes toxins into the bile system. The gallbladder is a sac that collects bile from the liver and discharges it into the intestinal tract through the common duct. If gallstone(s) or an inflammation impairs the flow of bile through the common duct, toxins will accumulate in the liver and re-enter the blood stream.

In a 1978 study, Breneman found that the common duct became inflamed from specific food allergies. This study revealed that the subjects also had these food allergies, in following percentages:
Eggs (93), Pork (64), Onions (52), Fowl (34.8), Milk (24.7), Coffee, (21.7), Oranges (19), Beans (14.5), Corn (14.5), Nuts (14.5), Apples (8.7), Tomatoes (7), Cabbages (5.8),

Peas (5.8), Peanuts (4.3), Spices (4.3), Fish (2.9), Rye (1.5), Medications (20.3), Other (42).

The main symptoms of gallbladder problems include: right upper quadrant pain (just under the rib cage), which may radiate from front to back; headaches; light colored stool; headaches; and nausea.

Water Deficiency

In addition to water being a source of toxic chemicals, a lack of adequate water can serve to decrease the amount of toxins eliminated.

The mechanism the body uses for eliminating toxins is to convert them from fat-soluble to water-soluble so they can be excreted by the kidneys. Drinking plenty of pure water will allow the body to rapidly excrete soluble waste products. Water is also important in moving material along the intestinal tract.

Water Calculator

Multiply weight in pounds by	0.5	______
Multiply minutes of exercise per day by	0.1	______
If pregnant, add	16	______
If breast feeding, add	24	______
If in a high altitude, add	8	______
If in a dry climate, add	8	______
Multiply number of caffeinated drinks per day by	4	______
Multiply number of alcoholic drinks per day by	8	______
If the weather very hot or very cold, add	16	______
If there is fever or diarrhea, add	8	______

Ounces of water needed per day – add totals		______
Quarts of water needed per day – divide totals by 32		______
8 oz. glasses of water needed per day – divide totals by 8		______

Emotional Stress

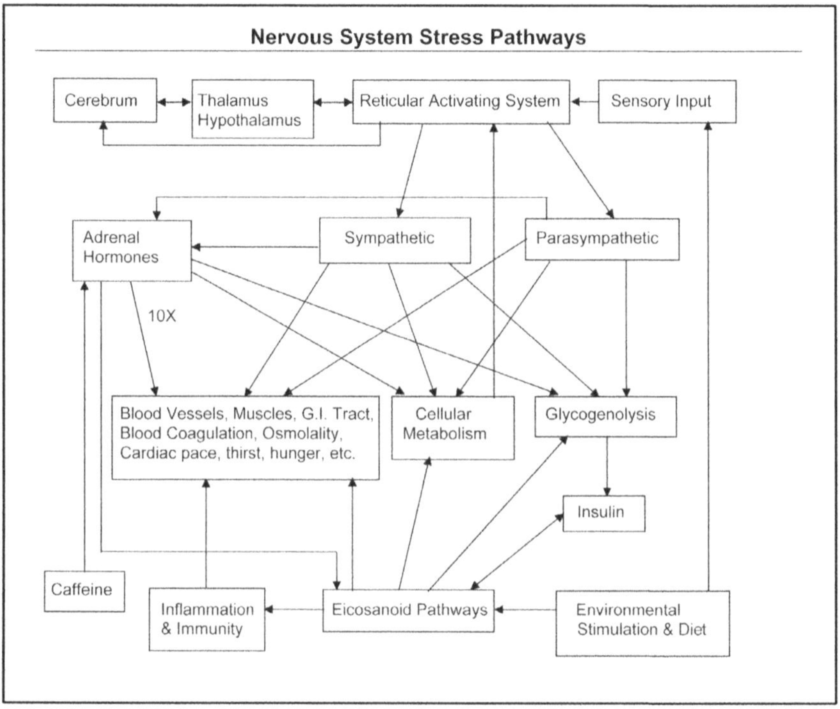

Coincidentally, the emotional center of the brain (the limbic system) is also the part of the brain that controls bodily function. Emotional stress leads to undesirable nervous system reactions, hormonal reactions and biochemical pathway changes throughout the body. Continuous emotional stress will have adverse effects on every cell in the body. It does not appear that nutrition or medicine can adequately compensate for the adverse effects of long-term hormonal, leukotriene, thromboxane, and inflammatory prostaglandin production. Consuming foods that are high in glycemic index and high in arachidonic acid, will significantly add to the adverse effects of emotional stress. It appears that the best and possibly the only method for eliminating the adverse effects of emotional stress is to reduce the emotional stress by various stress reduction methods.

The limbic system consists of the hypothalamus and the surrounding regions of the cerebral cortex, working together as a whole system. The hypothalamus controls all the autonomic nervous functions of the body such as, body temperature, osmolality of the body, thirst, hunger, body weight, heart rate, respiratory rate, gastrointestinal functions, etc. Basically, the hypothalamus controls all the bodily functions that don't require thought. The limbic system is also the center of emotions, where emotional memories are stored. Emotions have direct pathways that effect bodily functions through the limbic system. One common emotional reaction that stimulates a physiological reaction is sadness that stimulates the production of tears. The limbic system is also active in receiving and processing sensory signals for pain or pleasure.

Throughout the entire brain stem, there are areas of diffuse, short axon neurons that make multiple connections, known as the reticular formation or the reticular activating system. Consider viewing the reticular activating system as a kind of switching station that directs signals between the cerebrum and the autonomic nervous system.

The autonomic nervous system consists of the sympathetic nervous system and the parasympathetic nervous system. Sympathetic nervous stimulation dilates the pupils, increases heart rate and contractile force, constricts systemic blood vessels, increases blood coagulation and glucose, increases adrenal cortical secretion, increases mental activity, decreases kidney output, decreases peristalsis of the gut, increases strength and glycogenolysis of the skeletal muscles, etc. Glycogenolysis is the break down of glycogen to re-form glucose. The parasympathetic system effectively has the opposite effects on the same organs. Consider that the parasympathetic nervous system functions mainly to inhibit the sympathetic nervous system in a negative feedback loop. The activity of the autonomic nervous system can be controlled by the hypothalamus and the cerebrum. Many of the behavioral responses are affected by areas of the cerebrum sending signals to the hypothalamus, which sends signals through the reticular formation to the autonomic nervous system. The cerebrum can affect the entire autonomic nervous system severely enough to cause autonomic-induced disease such as gastric ulcers, constipation, heart palpitation, and heart attacks.

Excessive sympathetic stimulation may propagate a long-term hormonal effect on the body. For example, excessive sympathetic stimulation causes the adrenal medullae to produce large quantities of epinephrine (adrenaline) and norepinephrine. Normally, the ratio is 80% epinephrine and 20% norepinephrine. Epinephrine has almost the same effects as sympathetic stimulation. However, the epinephrine effects last about 10 times longer than the short-term sympathetic effects. Epinephrine has a stronger effect on cardiac activity, metabolism, and increased metabolic activities such as, glycogenolysis in the liver and muscle, and glucose release into the blood than norepinephrine. Norepinephrine has a stronger vasoconstrictive effect on the blood vessels than epinephrine. Both epinephrine and norepinephrine increase the activity of the heart, inhibit peristalsis in the gastrointestinal tract, dilate the pupils, etc.

Anxiety is an emotional reaction that causes sympathetic stimulation by the cerebrum stimulating the hypothalamus and the autonomic nervous system through the reticular activating system. Environmental stimulation such as traffic, loud noises, ordinary fluorescent lighting, computer cathode ray tube monitors, and many others, can constantly stimulate our sympathetic nervous system. Ordinary fluorescent lighting and cathode ray tube monitors and televisions, cause a flicker at 30 and 60 hertz, which cannot be detected by the human eye. However, this flicker can be detected by the brain causing the brain to become stimulated constantly by the flicker. Compact fluorescent bulbs with an electronic ballast (they usually have a regular light bulb base), do not flicker and have a full spectrum of colors. Full spectrum of colors in lighting has a similar effect on us as daylight. Liquid crystal display (LCD) computer monitors, which are also used in laptop computers, do not have a 30 or 60 hertz flicker.

Caffeine stimulates the adrenal medullae to produce large quantities of epinephrine and norepinephrine, which also leads to the previously discussed pathways.

Emotional stress, alcohol, and a tryptophan dose greater than two grams will activate the enzyme tryptophan oxygenase, which converts L-tryptophan into kynurenine, which then undergoes several conversions to become nicotinic acid (niacin), picolinic acid, and acetyl CoA. By converting much of the L-tryptophan into niacin and other compounds, there is less L-tryptophan available to be converted into serotonin. Low brain serotonin will result in insomnia and depression, depending on the level of serotonin in the brain. Low brain serotonin and low brain norepinephrine will result in migraine headaches. Low serotonin with high brain norepinephrine will result in mania.

Delta-6-Desaturase (D6D) is inhibited by adrenaline, steroids, and alcohol. D6D is the enzyme that converts lineolic acid into gamma-linolenic acid (GLA). GLA is converted into dihomo-gamma-linolenic acid (DGLA) by the enzyme, elongase. DGLA is the compound that produces the series 1 prostaglandins (PGE1). PGE1 is anti-inflammatory, vasodilative, blocks allergic response, improves nerve function, and enhances immune function.

Delta-5-Desaturase (D5D) is activated by insulin and inhibited by glucogon and eicosapentanoic acid. Insulin is produced in proportion to the glycemic index of foods and in response to the glycogenolysis, which results from increased sympathetic stimulation. For example, sugar and starch have high glycemic indexes. Consuming large amounts of sugar and starches will cause large amounts of insulin to be produced. Insulin also activates the activity of the enzyme HMG CoA reductase, which causes the liver to produce more cholesterol. D5D converts dihomo-gamma-linolenic acid into arachidonic acid. Arachidonic acid is found high in animal products, especially red meat. Arachidonic acid, mediated by the enzyme cyclooxygenase, is converted into series 2 prostaglandin and thromboxane. Series 2 prostaglandins and thromboxanes are pro-inflammatory, vasoconstrictive, cause platelet aggregation and clot formation, stimulates allergic response and renin secretion, suppresses immune function, inhibits insulin release, and inhibits norepinephrine release from synaptic junctions. Arachindonic acid mediated by the enzyme lipooxygenase is converted into hydroperoxyeicososatetraenoic acid and leukotrienes. Hydroperoxyeicososatetraenoic acid and leukotrienes are 1000 times more powerful than the prostaglandins, 1,000 to 10,000 times more inflammatory than histamine, vasoconstrictive, cause platelet aggregation and clot formation, stimulates allergic response and renin secretion, suppresses immune function, and stimulates secretion of mucus and air constriction. Aspirin and many other NSAID'S (Non Steroidal Anti-Inflammatory Drugs) will block the cyclooxygenase activity and consequently the pro-inflammatory pathways. However, they also block the anti-inflammatory pathways. Blocking the anti-inflammatory pathways can adversely affect immune function, nerve function, allergic reactions, and vasodilation. Eicosapentanoic acid and Docosahexanoic acid (fish oils, seed oils, mothers milk) produce series 3 prostaglandins, which are anti-inflammatory. Flax seed oil contains EPA and DHA. Flax seed oil also contains alpha-lenolenic acid, which can inhibit the delta-6-desaturase enzyme that is responsible for converting lineolic acid to gamma-linolenic acid.

Emotional stress also contributes to congestive bowel toxicity by tightening the bowel muscles and decreasing peristalsis.

Omega 6 Fatty Acid - Eicosanoid Pathways

Linoleic Acid (LA) C18:2w6 (sunflower, safflower, corn, sesame, seed and vegetable oils, legumes, mother's milk, etc.)

↓ Delta-6-Desaturase (D6D) (D6D is inhibited by adrenaline, Alpha-Linolenic Acid, and blocked by NSAID's, Steroids, & alcohol)
(D6D co-factors include: Vitamins A, B6, C, Folic acid, and Zinc, Copper, Magnesium)

Gamma-Linolenic acid (GLA) C18:3w6 (borage oil, evening primrose oil, black current oil, pumpkin, mother's milk)

↓ Elongase

Dihomo-Gamma-Linolenic Acid (DGLA) C20:3w6 → **Series 1: Prostaglandin (PGE1)**, (anti-inflammatory, vasodilative, blocks allergic response, improves nerve function, enhances immune function)

↓ Delta-5-Desaturase (D5D) (D5D is stimulated by Insulin, and inhibited by glucagon & EPA)

Arachidonic Acid C20:4w6 (animal products)

Cyclooxygenase → **Series 2: Prostaglandin (PGE2),** Thromboxane (A2), (pro-inflammatory, vasoconstrictive, tissue repair, platelet aggregation, clot formation, stimulates allergic response & renin secretion, increases glycogenolysis, suppresses immune function, inhibits insulin release, inhibits norepinephrine release from synaptic junction)
(blocked by NSAID's, Bioflavonoids, Ginger, Vitamin E EPA, Zinc

Lipoxygenase → **Hydroperoxyeicosatetraenoic acid, (HPETE), (HETE),** Leukotrienes (LT) - 1000x more powerful than PGE's, A's, 1,000-10,000x more inflammatory than histamine (pro-inflammatory, vasoconstrictive, tissue repair, platelet aggregation, clot formation, stimulates allergic response, suppresses immune function, stimulate secretion of mucus, airway constriction.)
(blocked by Bioflavonoids, Ginger, Vitamin E, Zinc, Selenium, EPA)

↑ Phospholipase
(blocked by Steroids & Vitamin E, stimulated by IgE allergic reactions)

Membrane Phospholipids

Nerve Stimulus → Norepinephrine release → PGE2
(inhibited by PGE2 at pre-synaptic junction) ←

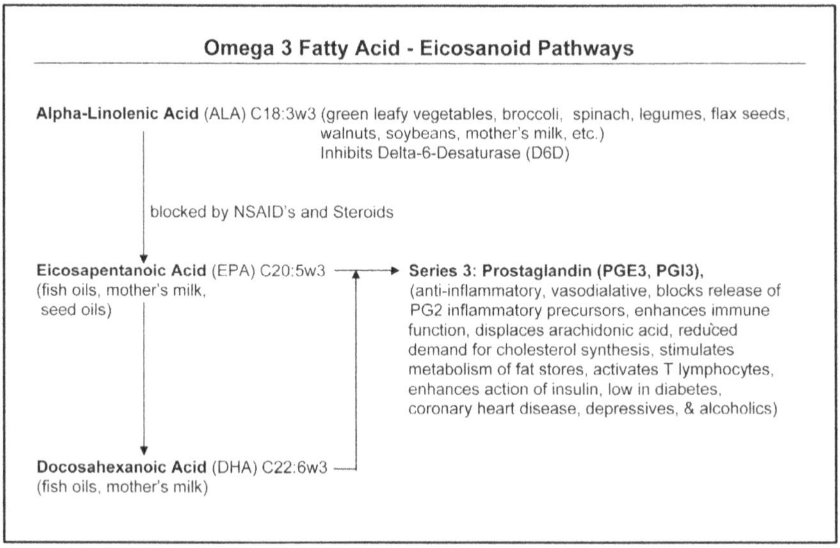

High Glycemic Index Foods

The endocrine system and the nervous system work together to regulate the appetite so that appropriate amounts of the appropriate foods are taken in. Refined white sugar has a high glycemic index and offsets this balance. This high-caloric dynamite explodes the pancreas and pituitary gland into hyper-secretion of hormones. Eating added sugar in various foods and drinks everyday chronically over-stimulates the pituitary and pancreas glands. The thyroid and adrenals also suffer. Many medical journals have implicated refined white sugar as a causative factor in: atherosclerosis, coronary heart disease, kidney disease, liver disease, shortening of life span, making blood platelets stick together, causing rise in serum triglycerides, and increasing the desire for coffee and tobacco.

Why is this important? When excess glucose enters the blood, excessive insulin is produced to transport the excess glucose to the fat cells for storage. Insulin increases the activity of a liver enzyme called HMG CoA reductase, which causes the liver to produce excessive cholesterol.

Cholesterol in the proper amount is necessary for many functions in the body, such as a major constituent of cell membranes, and hormones. Cholesterol becomes a problem only when there is an excess of it in the blood. This is why we want to avoid foods that have a high Glycemic Index.

Insulin increases the activity of an enzyme called delta 5 desaturase, which converts dihomogammalinolenic acid to arachidonic acid. Arachidonic acid produces vasoconstrictive and inflammatory eicosenoids, which lead to arteriosclerosis and cardiovascular disease. Arachidonic acid is also found in high levels in red meat and egg yolks.

Foods that contain higher amounts of fiber, will have a lower Glycemic Index. Fiber slows the uptake of sugar into the blood stream. Foods that have a high glycemic index will be broken down into glucose faster and therefore enter the blood stream faster, hence causing more insulin to be produced.

The glycemic index is a relative scale for classifying foods according to the blood sugar response that they cause. It measures how fast the carbohydrate of a particular food is converted to glucose and enters the blood. The glycemic index for a particular food may be different for different individuals.

The numbers used in the glycemic index are percentages with respect to a reference food. In this list, they are given with respect to glucose. For example, brown rice, which has a glycemic index of 58, raises blood sugar more than barley, which has a glycemic index of 26. A food is generally considered to have a high Glycemic Index if it is greater than 50 (1/2 of the value of glucose). Glycemic Index values of foods below are adjusted proportionately so that Glycemic Index of glucose is equal to 100.

Avoid eating sugar (sucrose) from this point forward. Fructose (the sugar in fruit) is an excellent substitute. Sugar (sucrose) has a glycemic index of 67. Fructose has a glycemic index of 23. Fructose is technically one-third the glycemic index of sucrose. However, since fructose is twice as sweet to the taste as sucrose, you will use half as much. The effective glycemic index of fructose becomes one-sixth that of sucrose. Also note that protein enriched pasta has a glycemic index of about half that of white pasta. Many pastas are labeled as "enriched" but not "protein enriched," which may relate to iron enriched not protein enriched – read the labels carefully.

Chapter 5 - Biochemical Pathways of Detoxification

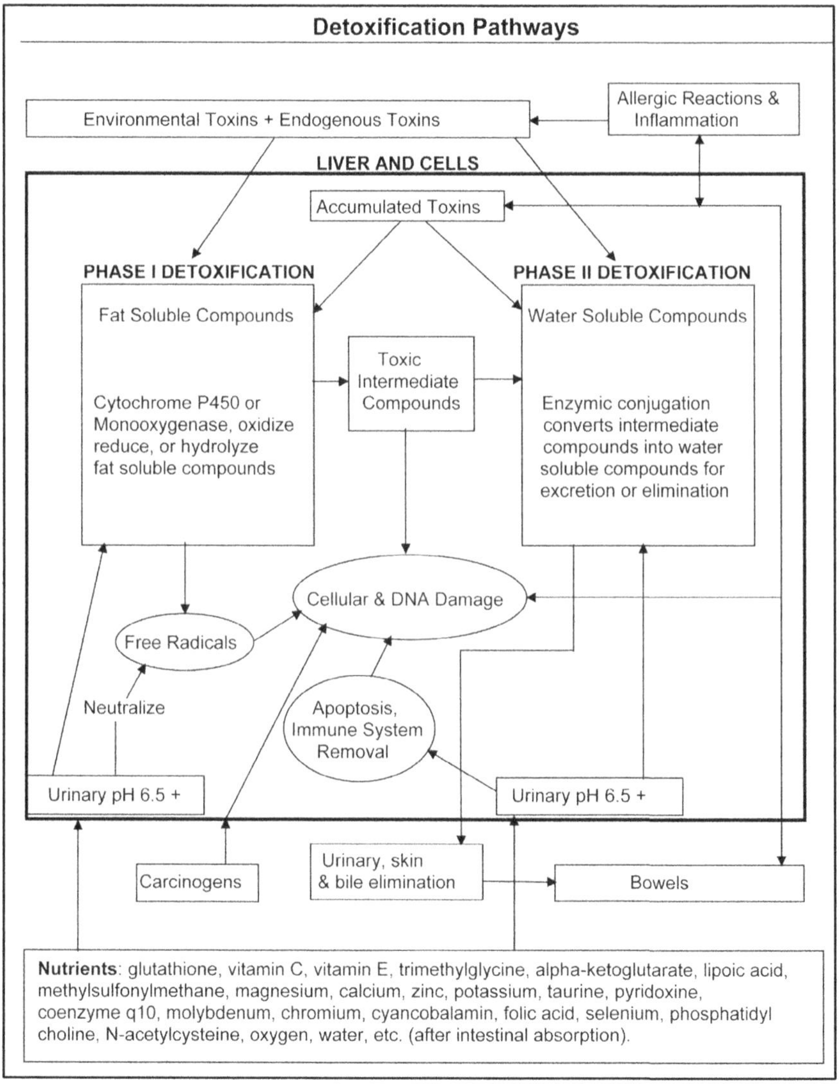
Detoxification Pathways
Environmental Toxins + Endogenous Toxins
Allergic Reactions & Inflammation
LIVER AND CELLS
Accumulated Toxins
PHASE I DETOXIFICATION
PHASE II DETOXIFICATION
Fat Soluble Compounds
Cytochrome P450 or Monooxygenase, oxidize reduce, or hydrolyze fat soluble compounds
Toxic Intermediate Compounds
Water Soluble Compounds
Enzymic conjugation converts intermediate compounds into water soluble compounds for excretion or elimination
Cellular & DNA Damage
Free Radicals
Neutralize
Apoptosis, Immune System Removal
Urinary pH 6.5 +
Urinary pH 6.5 +
Carcinogens
Urinary, skin & bile elimination
Bowels
Nutrients: glutathione, vitamin C, vitamin E, trimethylglycine, alpha-ketoglutarate, lipoic acid, methylsulfonylmethane, magnesium, calcium, zinc, potassium, taurine, pyridoxine, coenzyme q10, molybdenum, chromium, cyancobalamin, folic acid, selenium, phosphatidyl choline, N-acetylcysteine, oxygen, water, etc. (after intestinal absorption).

Damage to the cells from toxins is the major cause of many health problems. Toxicity from foreign chemicals (exotoxins) can cause damage to almost all cells of the body. Symptoms include: fatigue, headaches, neurological disorders, chemical sensitivities, immune dysfunction, and liver disorders. Food is often the main source of toxins. There are thousands of chemicals used by the food industry during processing and packaging. Many farmers use pesticides, which are passed along to us. In addition to these external sources of toxins, the body also produces toxins internally called, endotoxins resulting from digestion, immune system functions, stress, etc. Endotoxins may also be produced as the result of food allergies and sensitivities.

Increased intestinal permeability (leaky gut syndrome) can allow exotoxins to be absorbed into the blood stream along with antigens and microorganisms. Candida albicans overgrowth can cause an imbalance in the intestinal microflora (dysbiosis) and offset the immune response of the intestinal tract. Candida albicans can change to the mycel form and penetrate the intestinal wall, leaving behind microscope holes in the intestinal wall. Candida albicans also produce toxins called aldehydes. Supplementation with probiotics such as lactobacillus acidophilus and lactobacillus bifidus is important to keep candida albicans under control and maintain a balanced intestinal flora.

Congestive bowel toxicity can greatly increase the amount of toxins produced in the gastrointestinal track.

How does the body deal with toxins? Fat-soluble toxins are easily absorbed but poorly excreted. Often, they accumulate in the body and cause damage to tissues and organs. Fat-soluble chemicals are converted to water-soluble chemicals, primarily in the liver, and in some cells, in a two-step process so that the water-soluble toxins can be excreted by the urine, liver, and skin. The skin is a vitally important organ that eliminates toxins through perspiration.

During the first phase of detoxification, fat-soluble chemicals are converted into intermediate chemicals. As a result of this process, free radicals are also produced. The free radicals and the intermediate chemicals can cause damage to the cells. Adequate antioxidants must be present to detoxify these intermediate compounds produced during the first phase of detoxification. The first phase may also detoxify some chemicals directly without requiring a second phase conversion.

During the second phase, the intermediate chemicals are converted into water-soluble, chemicals, which are less toxic and easily excreted in the urine, bile, and skin.

It is now obvious why it is so important to avoid toxic chemicals from the environment. Drink uncontaminated water. Tap water should be filtered to remove lead, chlorine, heavy metals, and bacteria. It is also important to have an adequate supply of anti-oxidants to prevention cellular damage.

The ability of the liver to detoxify is determined by the availability of the appropriate nutrients and enzymes. An adequate supply of antioxidants is vitally important after the first phase of converting fat-soluble toxins, which produce free radicals. Reduced glutathione, superoxide dismutase, and catalase are the primary antioxidants used in the body to neutralize free radicals. Other antioxidants include: beta-carotene, vitamin E, vitamin C, selenium, N-acetylcysteine, Lipoic acid, and proanthocyanidins (grape seed extract). Vitamin and mineral cofactors required for cytochrome P-450 reactions include: riboflavin, niacin, magnesium, iron, and other trace minerals. Phytochemicals such as indoles from cruciferous vegetables and quercetin also help during the first phase of detoxification.

Other second phase conjugating agents include: amino acids such as glycine, cysteine, glutamine, methionine, taurine, glutamic acid, and asparatic acid.

Vitamin, mineral, and protein deficiencies will decrease the activity of the detoxification pathways. Fats and omega 6 polyunsaturated oils can promote the uptake of many chemical carcinogens. Olive oil (monounsaturated) and omega 3 polyunsaturated oils (EPA, DHA) have a neutral effect in promoting the uptake of carcinogens.

Cruciferous vegetables such as broccoli, cauliflower, brussel sprouts, watercress, and cabbage enhance the first phase of detoxification.

Garlic and onions contain flavonoid compounds, such as quercetin. Which diminish the mutation of many carcinogens.

Turmeric contains curcumin, which acts as an antioxidant and helps protect cells and DNA from free radical damage. Turmeric also acts as an anti-inflammatory agent.

As previously discussed, the detoxification process requires various nutrients to function. Without such nutrients in the cells, intermediate compounds can cause cellular and DNA damage. If the apoptosis system (cells self destruct if they are damaged) does not get the proper nutrients, the damaged cells can reproduce. If the immune system does not get the proper nutrients, the damaged cells can reproduce out of control causing cancer.

Getting the nutrients into the blood is only the first step. The nutrients must enter the cells in order to be available for use by the cells. In order for the nutrients to get into the cells, they must be transported though the cell membrane. When there is a lack of nutrients, particularly oxygen inside the cell, there is a build-up of lactic acid inside the cell. Excessive lactic acid damages the cell membrane transport mechanism and DNA. Lactic acid causes the cell to become acidic (lower pH). There is a weak correlation between intracellular pH and urine/saliva pH. The urine pH or saliva pH must be 6.5 or greater, which indicates the maximum amount of lactic acid in the cell, for the membrane transport mechanisms to function at peak performance.

Chapter 6 - Microorganisms that Damage Cell Membranes

Bacteria

Bacteria can produce phenylacetate, which is a potent neurotoxin. Bacteria can also produce tyramine, which is a potent vasoactive compound that directly displaces neurotransmitters, such as norepinephrine. This is often seen in migraine and depression.

Mild tyramine reactions can occur with approximately 6 mg of tyramine.

Severe reactions can occur with 10-25 mg tyramine of tyramine.

Approximate tyramine contents of food:

Cheddar cheese = 1.5 mg/g (42.5 mg/ounce)

Blue Stilton = 0.2 mg/g (5.6 mg/ounce)

Recently, more and more cases are appearing of patients who have an immune system reaction to Lactobacillus Acidophilus. In these cases, the stool analysis indicated zero acidophilus, while bifidus and other bacteria were normal.

A practitioner's first instinct may be to supplement with Lactobacillus Acidophilus to replenish the bacteria that is missing in the intestinal track. In some cases the reaction to Lactobacillus Acidophilus is subtle, while others have substantial reactions. These cases should be supplemented with bifidus bacteria.

Probiotic supplementation should be taken ONLY IN SMALL DOSES, not greater than 2 billion organisms because bacteria, friendly or unfriendly, produce tyramine. The larger the dose, the more tyramine that can be produced.

Tyramine Pathways

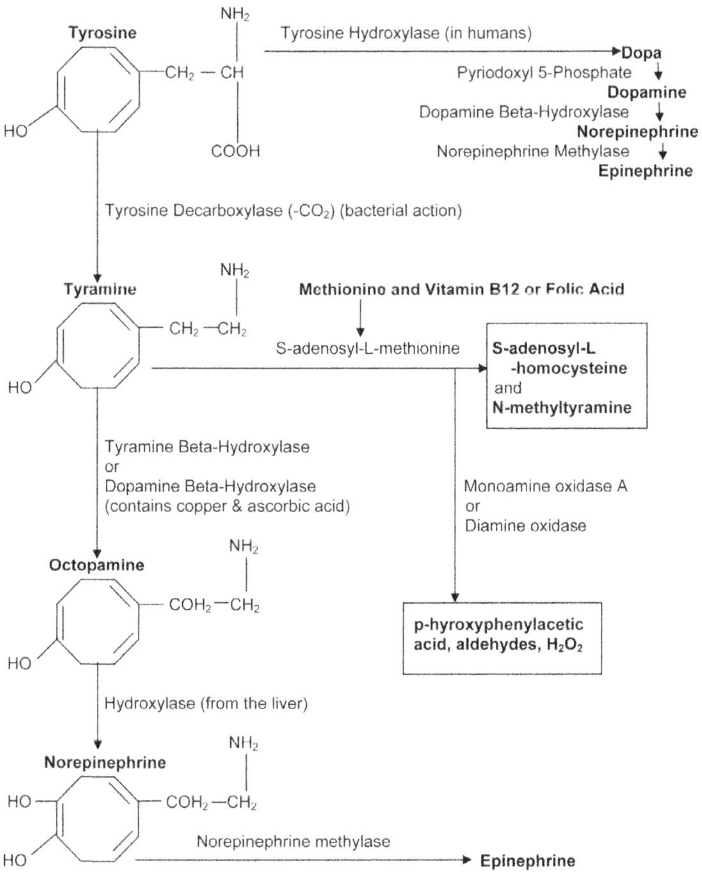

Tyramine is a potent vasoconstrictor and displaces neurotransmitters.
Octopamine is a potent vasoconstrictor in humans and neurotransmitter in insects.

The Cell

Cells are the basic living units of the body. Each organ is actually a conglomeration of many different cells held together by intercellular substances and structures. The cell membrane or cell wall normally keeps the internal parts together.

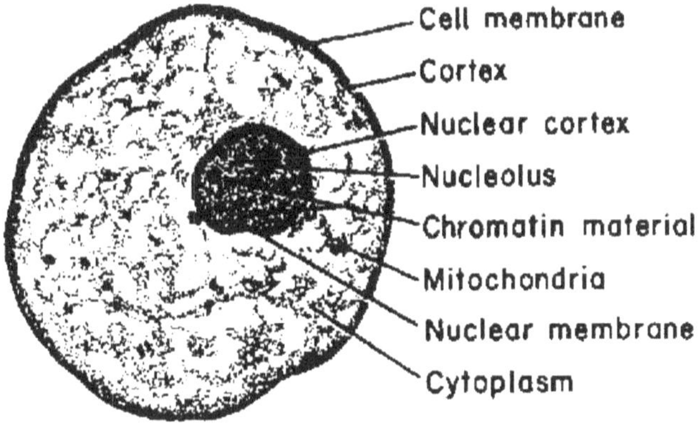

In the 21st Century a new breed of bacterial and fungi forms have appeared. Medicine is not yet equipped to diagnose these new types of microorganism or treat them.

Acquired Immunity

Acquired immunity is a special system that forms antibodies and sensitizes lymphocytes that attack and destroy the specific microorganisms or toxins.

Innate Immunity

Innate immunity results from general processes such as phagocytosis of invaders by the white blood cells and tissue macrophage system, destruction by the acid secretions of the stomach and by digestive enzymes, and resistance of the skin to invasion by organisms.

Antigens

Each toxin or type of microorganism has one or more specific chemical compounds in its structure that are different from all other compounds. These compounds are usually large polysaccharides or large lipoprotein complexes called antigens.

The Antigen-Antibody System

The antigen-antibody system is like a lock and key. An appropriately coded key must be made to fit in and turn the lock cylinder. Upon entry of a foreign antigen the lymphoid tissue macrophages phagocytize the antigen and then present it to adjacent lymphocytes, which produce antibodies that match the antigen.

Antibodies are gamma globulins called immunoglobulins and composed of polypeptide chains. Antibodies can inactivate an invader in several ways:

- Agglutination
- Precipitation
- Neutralization

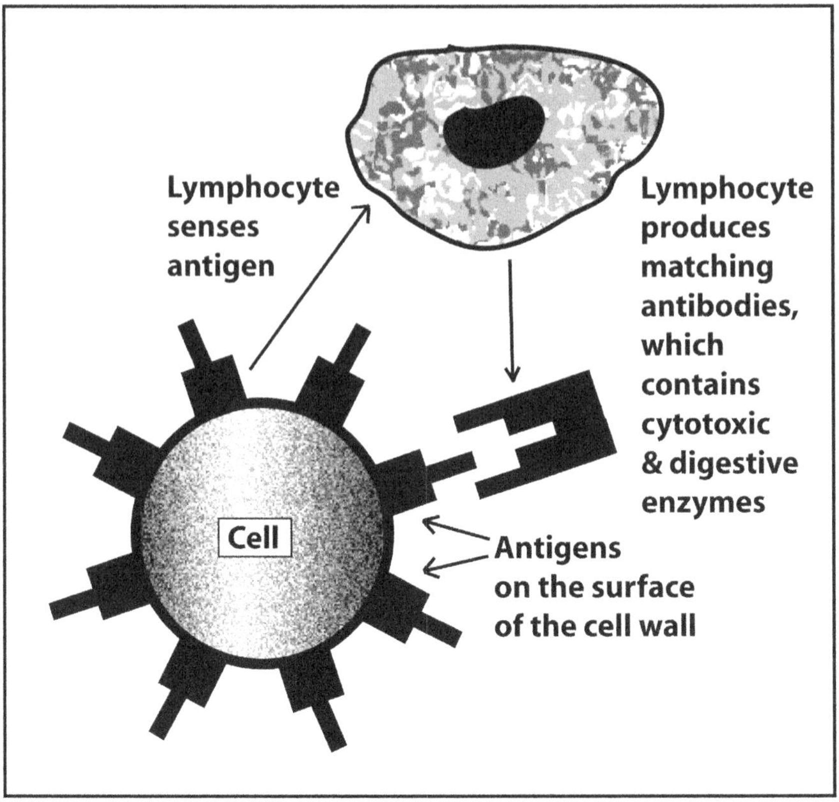

The antigen-antibody system worked well for thousands of years.

Now, we enter the 21st century...

21st Century Microbiology

The frequent use of antibiotics has spawned new forms of microorganisms.

Normally, the cell wall membranes of bacteria and fungi contain antigen codes, which are detected by the immune system. The immune system in turn produces antibodies to match the antigen of the bacteria or fungi. The antibodies attach to the microorganisms and destroy them.

These new forms of microorganisms are lacking complete cell wall membranes. The immune system will not produce antibodies because it didn't detect an antigen code. Nor will the immune system raise the body temperature, which is normally the first sign of infection.

Dr. Allocca, a medical research scientist, has been studying this phenomenon for more than 2 decades. At the beginning of this research, almost everyone responded with the comment:

"You cannot have an infection without fever."

The appearance of A.I.D.S patients who had systemic fungal infections and exhibited oral thrush without fever was the first clear evidence that there can be an infection without a fever.

We have a lot of progress in the past two decades. Cell wall deficient microorganisms are being recognized.

However, diagnosing their existence has been challenging since they don't produce antibodies that can be detected by normal blood tests.

Cell wall deficient microorganisms are responsible for many health disorders. Because they haven't been detected, these patients are usually labeled with chronic fatigue syndrome, fibromyalgia, and a host of other unidentifiable disorders.

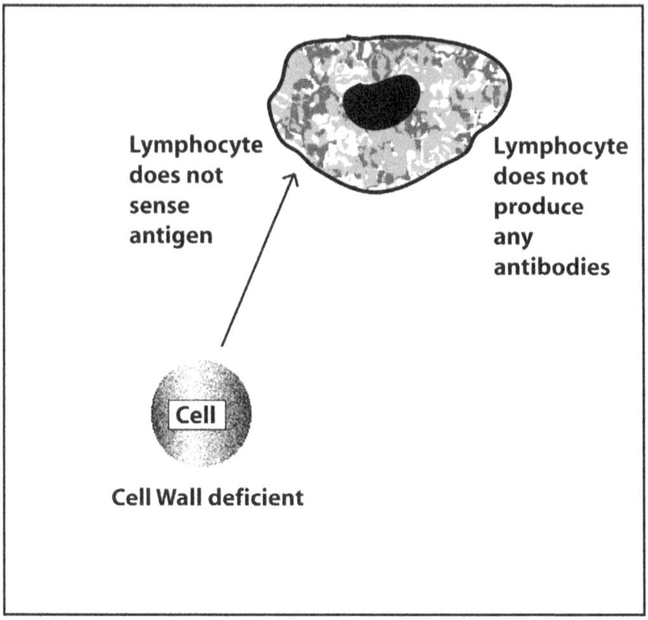

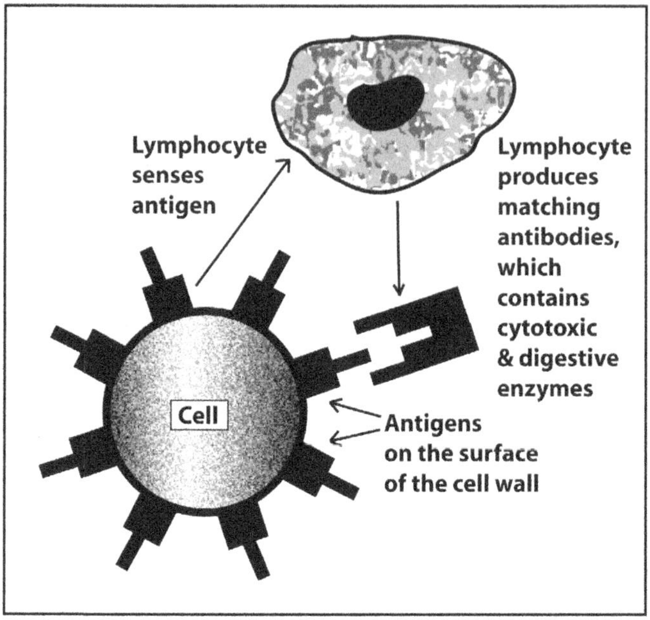
Lymphocyte
senses
antigen
Lymphocyte
produces
matching
antibodies,
which
contains
cytotoxic
& digestive
enzymes
Cell
Antigens
on the surface
of the cell wall

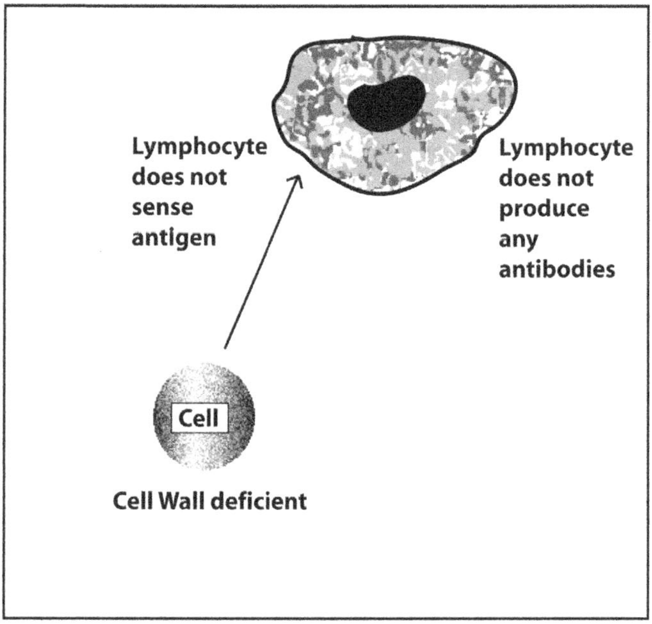
Lymphocyte
does not
sense
antigen
Lymphocyte
does not
produce
any
antibodies
Cell
Cell Wall deficient

L-form bacteria, also knows as L-phase bacteria, L-phase variants or cell wall deficient (CWD) bacteria, were discovered in 1935 by Emmy Klieneberger-Nobel, who named them L-forms after the Lister Institute in London in 1935.

L-form bacteria cannot reproduce in the cell wall deficient form. They must re-grow their cell wall in order to reproduce. It is at this point they are vulnerable to destruction by antimicrobials.

Identification

Cell wall deficient microorganisms are called L-forms, Cysts, and more. L-forms are small, gray, motile particles about 0.25 um in diameter. L-forms may appear like chylomicrons except they move rapidly around the slide under darkfield microscopy, which does not require staining and can sustain living blood for a period of time.

Some L-forms in the blood are normal. Substantial amounts of L-forms indicate a "hidden bacterial infection.

L-forms are cell wall deficient microorganisms, usually bacteria. L-forms are tiny, 0.25 um diameter, highly motile particles, in living blood as viewed under darkfield microscopy. Excessive L-forms indicate a hidden infection.

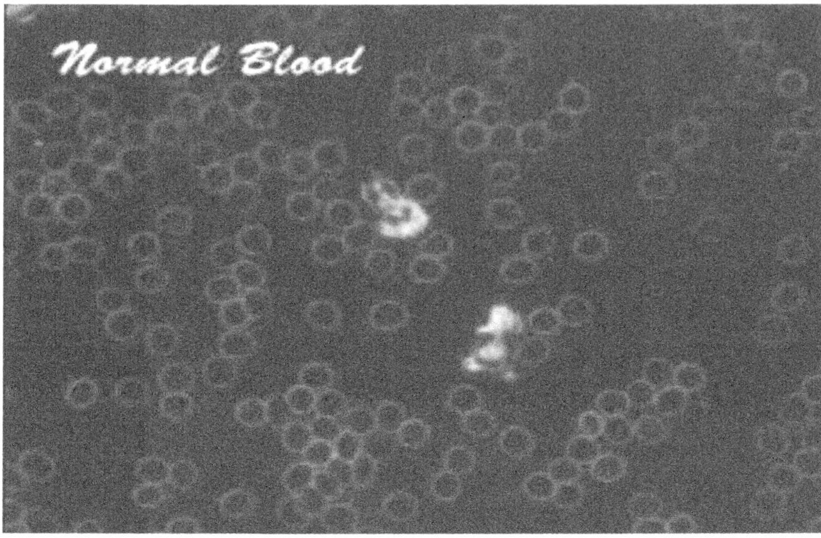
Normal Blood

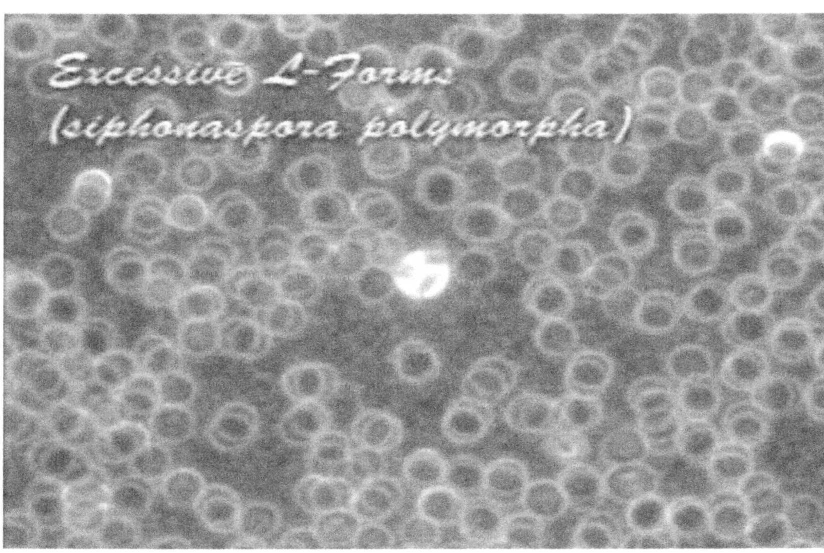
Excessive L-Forms
(siphonaspora polymorpha)

Fungi

Candida albicans is a common fungi that resides in the G.I. track, can also exist in cell wall deficient form. Often seen as large or larger than a RBC. Candida albicans can be identified under darkfield microscopy, even in the cell wall deficient form. One method is to stain the slide with a cellulose specific fluorescent stain. Another method is to visualize the growth of spores.

Symptoms

Fatigue
Headaches, including migraine
Depression
Muscle aches and pains
Joint pain and/or swelling
Abdominal pain
Alternating constipation and diarrhea
Abdominal bloating
Intestinal gas
Indigestion
Chemical sensitivities
Food allergies
Hypoglycemia
Premenstrual Tension
Endometriosis
Prostatitis
Vaginitis
Chronic dermatological infections or rashes
Acne

Inability to concentrate
Frequent mood shifts
Loss of memory
Lethargy
and more...

Roundworms

The family of Round Worms (Nematodes) include:

Ascariasis (Ascaris lumbricoides)
Cosmopolitan, more common in warm moist climates

Hookworm (Ancylostoma duodenale)
Temperate, warm moist climates

Theadworm - Strongyloidiasis (Stronyloides stercoralis)
Southern USA, moist tropics

Whipworm - Trichuriasis (Trichuris trichiura)
Warm, moist climates, Uncommon in USA

Enterobiasis (Enterobius vermicularis)
Cosmopolitan, especially in children

Round worm infections results from contaminated soil and raw vegetables

Chapter 7 - Biochemical and Biophysics Pathways of Cellular Metabolism

Phosphorus – Oxygen Double Bond

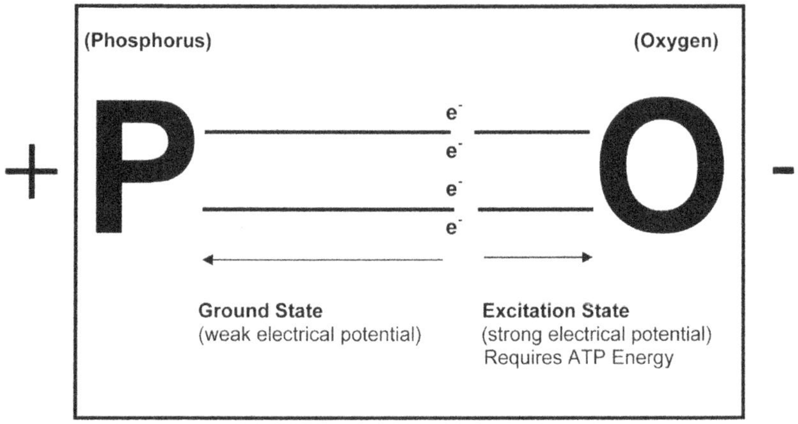

The phosphorus – oxygen double bond requires ATP energy to move Electrons closer to the oxygen molecule, which increases the electrical Potential of the bond to reach the excitation state, which is the point at Which, it transports all nutrients into the cell.

Alkaline cation transport at ground state: Cs^+, Rb^+, K^+, K.glucose

Alkaline cation transport at excitation state: Cs^+, Rb^+, K^+, Ba^{++}, Na^{++}, Li^+, Mg^{++}, K.glucose, H^2O, O_2

Aerobic Glycolysis (with oxygen)

$C_6H_{12}O_2$ (glucose) + 6 O_2 ⟶ $6H_2O$ + 6 CO_2 + 38 ATP

Anaerobic Glycolysis (without oxygen)

$C_6H_{12}O_2$ (glucose) ⟶ 2 $C_3H_6O_3$ (lactic acid) + 2 ATP

During anaerobic (without oxygen) glycolysis, there is a build up of lactic acid inside the cells, which damages the double bond and cellular DNA. An acid pH is a reflection of high lactic acid in the cell.

Oxygen is required for aerobic glycolysis to produce higher amounts of ATP for cellular metabolic energy and to bring the double bond to excitation state.

Potassium, with the help of insulin, can carry glucose into the cells. The intake of large quantities of potassium can provide more potassium than is needed for glucose transport supplying some free potassium, which makes the cell more alkaline, thereby neutralizing lactic acid.

Cesium and Rubidium can be used to alkalize and consequently neutralize the lactic acid in the cells. Caution should be taken with a dosage because they are both potent stimulants, which can cause anxiety and sever stomach pain. Cesium and Rubidium are available in the form Cesium Chloride and Rubidium Chloride. An alternative would be to use calcium citrate, potassium citrate, and magnesium citrate.

Membrane Transport

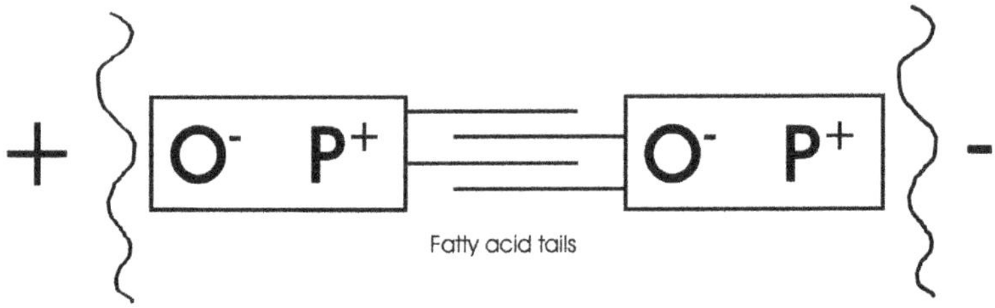

Alkaline cation transport at ground state: Cs^+, Rb^+, K^+, K.glucose

Alkaline cation transport at excitation state: Cs^+, Rb^+, K^+, Ba^{++}, Na^{++}, Li^+, Mg^{++}, K.glucose, H^2O, O_2

At excitation state (with oxygen): Glucose ($C_6H_{12}O_2$) $\xrightarrow[6\ O_2]{\text{aerobic}}$ $6H_2O + 6\ CO_2 + 38$ ATP

At excitation state (without oxygen): Glucose ($C_6H_{12}O_2$) $\xrightarrow{\text{anaerobic}}$ $2\ (C_3H_6O_3) + 2$ ATP
(lactic acid)

Cancer Pathways

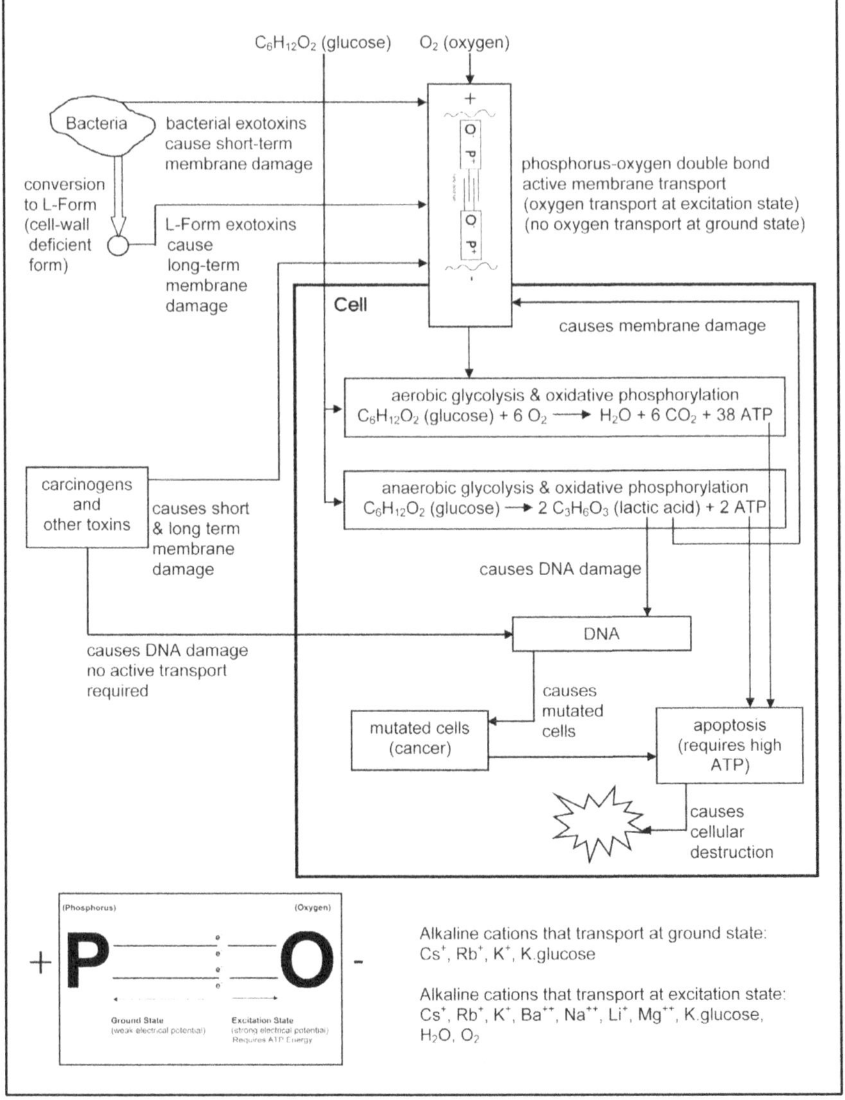

Oxygen deficiency in cells, results primarily from inadequate mechanism of transport through the cell membrane rather than the amount of oxygen in the blood, except in cases where athletic activity does not supply enough oxygen to the blood. Energy is produced through the glycolytic pathway. In glycolysis, glucose is converted to glucose-6-phosphate, then to glycogen and/or pyruvate and 2 molecules of ATP (energy). Glycolysis does not require any oxygen (anaerobic). In the absence of oxygen, the process of oxidation and phosphoryation consumes the cells supply of NAD^+ (nicotinamide adenine dinucleotide). NADH can be reoxidized by converting pyruvate to lactate in the presence of lactic dehydrogenase (LDH), which favors the conversion of pyruvate to lactate. In the presence of oxygen, pyruvate undergoes oxidative decarboxylation whereby pyruvate + NAD^+ + CoA is converted to acetyl CoA + NADH + CO_2. Acetyl CoA is the beginning of the Krebs (Citric acid) cycle, which produces 38 molecules of ATP (energy), carbon dioxide, and water, through oxidative phospholoryation (aerobic). The five coenzymes needed for these reactions are thiamin pyrophosphate, lipoic acid, CoA, FAD, and NAD^+. The four water-soluble vitamins needed are thiamin, riboflavin, nicotinic acid, and pantothenic acid. If there is a lack of oxygen in the cell, there will be a build up of lactic acid, which can dramatically alter the pH of the cell to be more acidic. In the acidic environment, enzymes from lysosomes within the cell are released and react with the acidic surroundings, which may prevent the membrane double bonds from reaching higher excitation levels and eventually damage the cells DNA.

The rate of glucose transport into the cells increases to as much as ten times in the presence of insulin. Excessive amounts of insulin, which can occur when consuming high glycemic index foods, can create excessive amounts of glucose in the cells. Without adequate, oxygen in the cells, there can be a build up of lactic acid, which can dramatically alter the pH of the cell to be more acidic. In the acidic environment, enzymes from lysosomes within the cell are released and react with the acidic surroundings, which may prevent the double bonds from reaching higher excitation levels and eventually damage the cells DNA.

The most important part of the cell membrane is the phosphorous and oxygen double bond (P=O). Four electrons are closer to the oxygen atom than the phosphorous atom, which creates an electrical potential ($P^+ = O^-$). This electrical potential can cause cations to enter or leave a cell. The cell membrane contains a double layer of these bonds, connected by fatty acid tails, creating complex pumping action in and out of the cells. The strength of the attraction depends upon the excitation level of double bond in the cell membrane. At the lowest excitation level (ground state) of the double bond, it produces the smallest electrical potential across the cell membrane. At the ground state, the cell membrane can only transport $Cesium^+$, $Rubidium^+$, and $Potassium^+$ alkaline cations into the cell. Therefore, the membrane can transport primarily water and glucose. In the ground state the cell membrane will have great difficulty in transporting oxygen into the cells. As previously described, there will be a build up of lactic acid, which changes the cellular pH. The energy required to increase the excitation level of the double bond is produced within the cell. At the higher energy levels, the four electrons of the double bond are pulled farther away from the phosphorus atom, which results in higher electrical potentials across the cell membrane, which results in greater transport of molecules into the cell. At the high excitation levels of the double bond, the cell membrane can transport water, glucose, oxygen, and other nutrients into the cell.

Carcinogens are chemicals with certain electrical properties that coat the cell membrane, which prevent the higher excitation levels of the double bonds, which results in mostly water and glucose being transported into cells. The cells become deficient in oxygen and other nutrients. The cancer process begins with the loss of approximately one third of the oxygen transport into the cell. Anaerobic metabolism causes a build up of lactic acid within the cell, which dramatically changes the pH of the cell to acidic. In the acidic environment, enzymes from lysosomes within the cell are released and react with the acidic surroundings, which may prevent the double bonds from reaching higher excitation levels. The acidic environment will eventually damage the DNA within the cells resulting in a loss of the usual genetic controls whereby cellular size and shape are no longer regulated.

The normal pH range for cells is about 7.3 to 7.4. Death occurs when the blood pH falls to 7.0 or rises to 8.0. Intracellular pH ranges from 6.0 to 7.4. If the cell drops below 6.0 or rises above 8.0, the cell dies. Normal cells can maintain this narrow range of pH through the pH buffering system, which consists of sodium bicarbonate ($NaHCO_3$) and carbonic acid (H_2CO_3) in the same solution. In the intracellular fluid, there is little sodium bicarbonate and the bicarbonate ion occurs primarily as potassium and magnesium bicarbonate. There are also phosphate and protein buffering systems. In the low excitation state, the double bonds may not be able to transport enough molecules to significantly change the pH of a very acidic cellular environment.

If the normal buffering system cannot elevate the pH of a cell, various elements can be used to accomplish this task. Molecules may lose electrons in water becoming positively charged ions called cations. Cations attract negatively charged ions called anions. Cations also raise the pH of the environment. Peroxides, water, glucose, amino acids, and various energy molecules are electrically neutral overall, but have positive and negative charges in various regions. Depending upon the strength of the attraction, these molecules can react with various elements. Cesium Cs^+ has a very weak attraction for negative charges and does not combine with many molecules. Its association appears to be limited to three water molecules ($Cs.3H_2O$). Rubidium is the second weakest element and appears to be limited to five water molecules ($Rb.5h_2O$). Potassium is the third weakest element and appears to be limited to seven water molecules ($K.7H_2O$) or glucose (potassium/glucose). Cesium is the most active cation and has the least association with most molecules. Therefore, it is the first choice that may be used to alter cellular pH without adverse reaction. Rubidium is the next element of choice. Raising the pH of the cells neutralizes the acidic lysosomal enzymes. Vitamins A and C attach to cell membranes and increase the transport of cesium and rubidium into the cells. Zinc and selenium form double bonds with oxygen and also increase the transport of cesium and rubidium into the cells. Populations such as the Hopi and Navajo, who have high levels of rubidium and potassium in their soil, have the lowest cancer rates.

The strength of alkaline elements are (from strongest to weakest): cesium, rubidium, potassium, barium, sodium, calcium, lithium, and magnesium.

The transport of cations at ground state are (from minimum potential double bond gradient to maximum potential double bond gradient required): cesium, rubidium, potassium.

The transport of cations at excited state are (from minimum potential double bond gradient to maximum potential double bond gradient required): cesium, rubidium, potassium, barium, sodium, calcium, lithium, magnesium.

Cesium and rubidium are potent stimulants. Caution should be exercised when using them to raise pH and neutralize lactic acid. They can cause hyperactivity, irritability, and loss of temper.

Potassium, with the help of insulin can carry glucose into the cell. The intake of large quantities of potassium can provide more free potassium than is needed for glucose transport supplying some free potassium, which makes the cell more alkaline, thereby neutralizing the lactic acid. The minimum required daily amount (RDA) for potassium is 2,000 mg.

Bibliography

Berkow, R., et al, The Merck Manual, Sixteenth Edition, Merck Research Laboratories, New Jersey, 1992.

Brown, J.E., The Science of Human Nutrition, Harcourt Brace, New York, NY; 1991

Dyerberg et al, Eicosapentanoic acid and prevention of thrombosis and arteriosclerosis, Lancet, vol. 2, 1978.

Fernstrom, MH, et al, Brain tryptophan concentrations and serotonin synthesis remain responsive to food consumption after the ingestion of sequential meals, Am J Clin Nutr, PA, 1995.

Fisher, Richard B., Ph.D., A Dictionary of Body Chemistry, Paladin, Granada, NY, 1983.

Fozard, JR, The 5-hydroxytryptamine-nitric oxide connection: the key link in the initiation of migraine, Arch. Int. Pharmacodyn Ther, Switzerland, 1995.

Ginsburg, I., Phagocytosis of Candida albicans enhances malignant behavior of murine tumor cells, Science, December 1987.

Guyton, A., Textbook of Medical Physiology, sixth edition, W.B. Saunders Company, 1981.

Harper, H., Mayes, P., Review of physiological chemistry, Lange med. pub., vol. 182, 1979.

Harrison's Principles of Internal Medicine, McGraw-Hill, New York, 1974.

Jaffe, RM, Eosinsophia-Myalgia Syndrome Caused by Contaminated Tryptophan, Int. J. Biosocial Med Research, USA 1989.

Lehninger, A., Principles of Biochemistry, Worth Publishers, Inc., New York, 1982.

Loebel-Noack et al, Influence of different dairy regimens upon the composition of the human fecal flora, Prog. Ed. Nutr. Sci., 1983.

Levine et al, Oxidants/antioxidants and chemical hypersensitivities, Biosocial research, vol 4, 1983.

Krause, M.V., Mahon, K., Eds., Krauses Food and Nutrition Diet Therapy 8th Edition, W.B. Saunders, Philadelphia, PA, 1992.

Michelson, D, et al, An eosinophilia-myalgia syndrome related disorder associated with exposure to L-5-hydroxytryptophan, J Rheumatol, 1994.

Murray, Michael and Pizzorno, Joseph, Eds. 1991, Encyclopedia of Natural Medicine. Rocklin, CA; Prima Publishing

Orten, J., Neuhaus, O., Human Biochemistry, tenth edition, The C.V. Mosby Co., St. Louis, 1982.

Pattichis, K, et al, 5-Hydroxytryptamine release from platelets by different red wines: implications for migraine, London, UK, 1995.

Pollock, M., Alcohol and the nervous system, New Zealand Medical Journal, January 1974.

Physician's Handbook, Krupp, M, et al, Lange Medical Publications, Los Altos, California, 1982.

Reddy et al, Natural antibiotic activity of L. Acidophilus and Bulgaricus, Cult. Dairy Prod. J., vol. 18, 1983.

Shahani, K., Ayebo, A., Role of dietary lactobacilli in gastrointestinal microecology, The American Journal of Clinical Nutrition, November 1989.

Shils, Maurice E., Olson, James A., Shike, Moshe; Modern Nutrition in Health and Disease, 8th Edition, Lea and Febiger, 1994.

Tapple, A., Will antioxidant nutrients slow the aging process?, Geriatrics, vol. 23, 1968.

Virkkunen, M, Low brain serotonin turnover rate (low CSF 5-HIAA) and impulsive violence, J Psychiatry Neurosci, Finland, 1995.

Wang, W, Intensity dependence of auditory evoked potentials is pronounced in migraine: an indication of cortical potentiation and low serotonergic neurotransmission, Neurology, Belgium, 1996.

Watts, H., Handbook of Medical Treatment, Seventeenth Edition, Jones Medical Publications, California, 1983.

Weiller, C, et al, Brain stem activation in spontaneous human migraine attacks, Nat Med, Germany, 1995.

Made in the USA
Monee, IL
04 November 2026

67378674R00046